Chakra Balancing

Made Simple and Easy

Michael Hetherington
(L. Ac, Yoga Teacher)

Disclaimer

All material in this book is provided for your information only and may not be construed as medical advice or instruction. No action or inaction should be taken based solely on the contents of this information; instead, readers should consult appropriate health professionals on any matter relating to their health and well-being.

The information and opinions expressed here are believed to be accurate, based on the best judgment available to the authors, and readers who fail to consult with appropriate health authorities assume the risk of any injuries. The publisher is not responsible for errors or omissions.

About the Author

Michael Hetherington is a qualified acupuncturist, health practitioner and yoga teacher based in Brisbane, Australia. He has a keen interest in mind-body medicine, energetic anatomy, nutrition and herbs, lifestyle design, yoga nidra and Buddhist style meditation. Inspired by the teachings of many he has learnt that a light-hearted, joyful approach to life serves best.

Other Titles by Author:

How to Do Restorative Yoga

The Little Book of Yin

How to Learn Acupuncture

Moving From Our Head to Our Heart

The Art of Muscle Testing

Table of Contents

Introduction

Chakra balancing is a simple, safe, effective, non-invasive, and super easy healing technique that anyone can practice — anytime, anywhere. It is free to practice, all you need is an intention to help or heal, and your hand or arm.

Chakra balancing is an ancient healing art from the yogic traditions of India. There are elements of chakra balancing in Chinese medicine and traditional Japanese medicine, and these days it is also used in modern healing applications like applied kinesiology.

We will also discuss what it is not. It is non-religious and it is not an occult practice. There is no secret to it, no hidden codes or agendas, no special formulas or magic involved. It is simple, easy, and free to practice, and because we are all made up of energy, it is available to us all — it is universal. You can even do it with animals or any being that has a spinal column.

There is no harm that can come from chakra balancing. If the intent is to help, heal and support another being (or ourselves), then this intention acts like a prayer allowing a powerful energy to come through us. The practice of chakra balancing has a very positive effect on one's health and general well-being no matter what their condition.

How Does it Work?

We are energetic beings. We are gifted to carry an intelligent electromagnetic energy field around our bodies, which fuels, sustains and protects our physical form, as well as feeding and fuelling our mental and emotional states. It is like a complex grid of electricity, also known as an "auric" field. In the modern world this grid or energy often gets disturbed and scrambled by outside influences. It can also become dysfunctional by internal energy blocks and stagnations, therefore it is important to keep our chakras spinning and functioning well. This is a super simple technique that uses our arms and hands to encourage the natural "spinning" flow of the chakras.

What are Chakras?

The word chakra means "vortex" or "energy centre" or "wheel". There are seven in the yogic system, and three main ones in the Oriental system. There are also minor chakras that exist in the palms, feet, and behind the knees, to name just a few. The seven chakras are closely associated with the endocrine glands, better known in biomedical anatomy.

Personally, I understand chakras to be like portals where subtle energies and information from higher planes of existence, like the quantum field, are funneled through to us. The chakras then distribute this information and energy through the meridians that run through the body like a complex river and irrigation system. These subtle energies influence matter and denser forms of reality, and this is where our experience of our dense physical bodies comes in.

Another way of describing it is that the nervous system, the brain and the endocrine glands act as receivers of this information, and, when triggered, secrete hormones into the body which instruct and dictate cellular activity. If the chakras and meridians are not functioning well, the nervous system, brain, and endocrine glands receive misinformation, and therefore secrete the incorrect mix of hormones so the cells start acting strangely. The body gets confused, physiology on all levels starts breaking down, the organs start suffering, and our psychological function becomes impaired.

The chakras also interact and draw in energy from our environments and from other beings. They draw in this energy for a variety of reasons — to experience, to learn, to assimilate, to entrain (synchronize), to nourish and to heal.

Our chakras spin both in clockwise and counterclockwise directions. The chakras are a complex system of energy transformation; a similar complexity to that of fractal geometry. One description is that the chakras are made up of discs, and the outer disc spins in a clockwise direction, the next disc spins in a counterclockwise direction, and so forth. Also, from my experience, men's chakras tend to have a greater clockwise than counterclockwise spin, and women have a greater counterclockwise than clockwise spin. The clockwise direction may symbolize "yang" and counterclockwise may symbolize "yin". Please note that both yin and yang are present in all things.

Signs and Symptoms of Chakra Dysfunction

- Headaches

- Poor digestion, bloating, distension, constipation, diarrhea, gas, etc.

- Cloudy mind; finding it hard to think

- Consistent feelings and thoughts of being lost in life and confused; depression

- Poor breathing and circulation

- Hip, knee, and ankle problems

- Uncoordinated movement

- Difficulty connecting with others; occasional inappropriate behavior

- Inability to express feelings to others

- Talking too much or not enough

- Tight or restricted feeling in throat; hoarse voice

- Getting sick easily; poor immune system

- Bad temper; frustration; irritability

- Inability to experience joy, laughter, or silliness easily; being too serious

- Stiff body; tight muscles; musculoskeletal aches and pains

- Sore, dry and irritated eyes; eye problems; blurry

vision

- Anxiety & anxiety attacks; nervous disorders

Bad Habits and How
They Affect the Chakras

In the ideal situation our chakras are all spinning and humming along in a balanced way. When they are all working this way, they support and nourish each other. There is an "ease" to life; a clear and balanced mind, and a good digestive system.

When a chakra goes out of balance it will eventually have an effect on the other chakras, most likely the chakras either just below or above the affected chakra.

When we have a chakra that is depleted, it finds its energy by adding some kind of stimulant or intoxicant that we put into the system, or by drawing energy from another chakra.

People who are out of balance in their chakras can also take energy from other beings that don't have the ability or capacity not to give over the energy because their overall system is deficient. This is common in dominating- and passive-based relationships.

Anything that essentially brings you out of balance can affect the function of your chakras. Usually dysfunction is caused by overactivity, overuse, overstimulation, or on the other end of the spectrum of stagnation, laziness and lack of movement or action.

The Technique

Balancing All the Chakras on Yourself

You can do this to yourself, or on somebody else if they give you consent. It's a great thing to do before a meeting, or giving a class, or before any event where you need to be at your best.

This can be done sitting or standing. I have supplied some photos to show you both ways.

1. Bring the most dominant hand down to the base chakra and start making circles in a clockwise motion for about 10 – 15 circles. If you can imagine a clock face placed on the front of your body, this will give you the idea and visual of a clockwise motion and a counterclockwise motion. Also, don't worry too much if you can't get the clockwise and counterclockwise thing worked out; it doesn't really matter. Just do one way and then the other…

Base chakra ~ clockwise

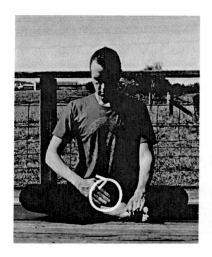 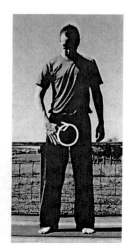

2. After you have done your circles, just shake your hand off, bring it back to base chakra position, and start going in a counterclockwise direction for about ten cycles (opposite direction as before).

Base chakra ~ counterclockwise

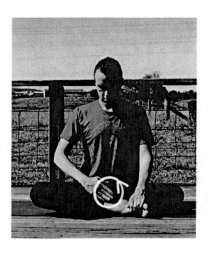 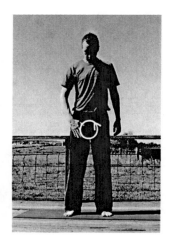

3. Again, at the end of doing your circles, shake off the hand. Then go to the sacral chakra and start making clockwise circles for 10 – 15 circles.

Sacral ~ clockwise

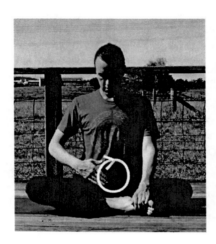 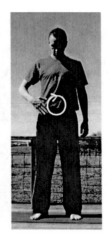

4. After you have done your clockwise circles, shake off your hand and do about ten counterclockwise circles on the sacral chakra.

Sacral ~ counterclockwise

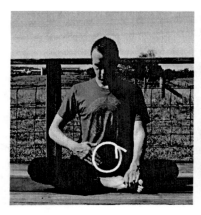 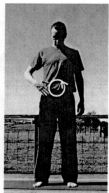

5. Continue all the way up to the top of the head, first going to each chakra and spinning clockwise 10 – 15 times. Then, shake off your hands; go counterclockwise for ten circles; shake off your hands and go up to next chakra.

Solar plexus ~ clockwise

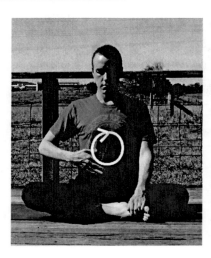 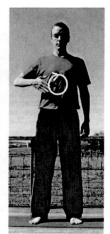

Solar plexus ~ counterclockwise

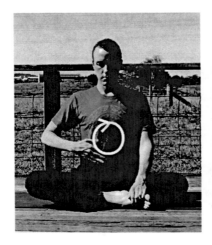
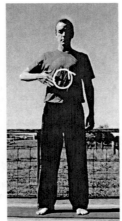

Heart chakra ~ clockwise

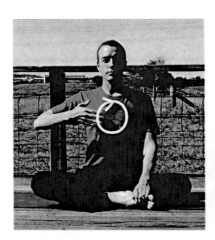
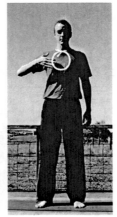

Heart chakra ~ counterclockwise

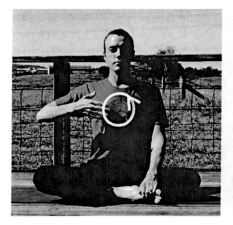 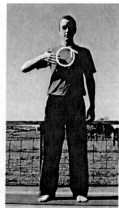

Throat chakra ~ clockwise

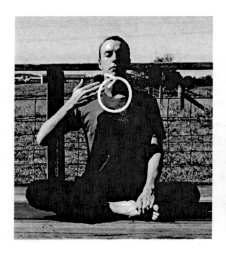 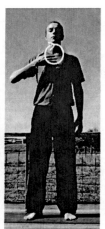

Third eye ~ clockwise

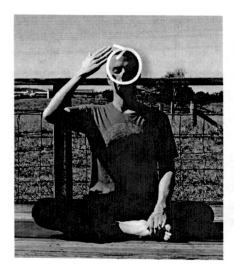 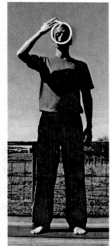

Third Eye ~ counterclockwise

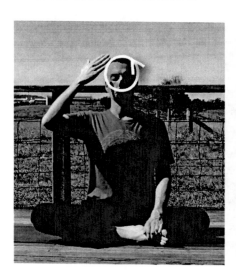 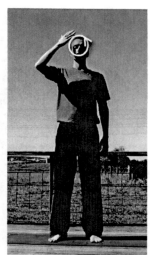

Crown ~ clockwise

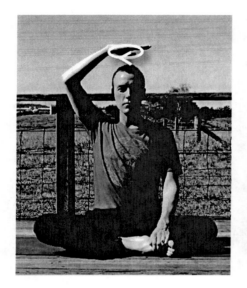 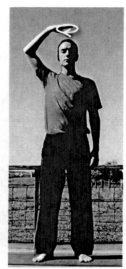

6. When you get to the crown chakra, the circles are more like you are tracing a crown just above the top of your head. As with the other chakras, again circle clockwise first and then counterclockwise.

If you get confused, don't worry; just do one way and then the other.

Crown ~ counterclockwise

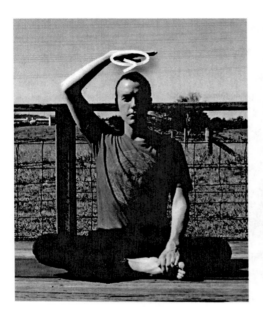 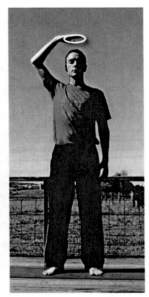

7. When completed, rest your arms, take a breath in, and relax. You are done. Take a sip of water. How do you feel now?

Balancing the Chakras on Somebody Else

Balancing the chakras on somebody else is pretty much the same as doing it on yourself, but they get to relax and rest while you do the work to balance them out.

1. Get the person (or yourself) to lie in a supine position. (A reclining chair or standing can also work.)

2. Both take a breath, and relax the body on the exhale.

3. You can check for any malfunctioning chakras using a few methods, or if you have time, you can spin all the chakras if you like; both are good options. To locate any dysfunction, try asking the person: "What part of the body do you feel the most? Do you have any pain or discomfort in your body, and if so, where is it?" Or, if they have the very common slumped-over posture, where the belly area is compressed and the shoulders and head are forward, then you can go straight to sacral, solar plexus, or heart to begin. Or you could try muscle testing (more on this later).

4. Simply bring your palm above the chakra in the area of focus and begin circling your hand and arm in a counterclockwise direction, like spinning a vinyl record on a record player. You can circle your hand close to the body to begin with; there is no need to touch the body with this technique. You can then draw the palm away from the body while continuing to

circle it. You can vary the distance from the body as much as you like or feel is appropriate. Most people feel warmth, or something like a dense, misty air with their palms while spinning. Spin for 1 – 5 minutes.

5. Next, shake your hands off, rub them together just to neutralize any electrical charge, and begin spinning in the same area, this time in a clockwise direction. Again, you can vary the distance from the body as you much as you like and feel is appropriate. Spin for 1 – 3 minutes (usually a little less than counterclockwise).

6. Now you can focus on the next chakra that has come to your attention, either through questioning or muscle testing. Repeat steps 4 – 5.

7. Repeat as many times as necessary to get all the chakras spinning well.

8. Finish by taking a breath and both drinking a sip of water.

Chakra Genetics

It is important to understand that every one of us has a predisposition to have certain strengths and potential weaknesses within our chakras. This can be likened to our genetic makeup and constitution. Therefore, every person or being usually has 1 – 3 chakras that are strong and dominant in their overall makeup, and this can reflect in the overall personality of the person. It's a good idea to learn what your strong and weak chakras are so that you can be more proactive in developing them accordingly.

Develop your ability to sense these areas in your body. What feels sluggish and what feels clear? Sluggish feelings almost always indicate the area is not functioning well, and the chakras will be out. Clear areas indicate that the area is working well and is "switched on".

I recommend focusing on your weak chakras first to get them functioning at optimal levels. When the weaker ones are functioning well, the stronger chakras will be energetically supported and will usually develop themselves.

Sometimes people use their genetics as an excuse for always being sick or unwell, and sometimes it's just a copout. Genetics do play a part in our health and evolutionary journey, but I firmly believe that genetic weaknesses can be overcome if one is persistent and genuine in their endeavors to evolve and reach their highest potential. With proper diet, ongoing energetic balancing, and taking the time and effort to develop your courage and creative potential, you can overcome and clear out any genetic weakness from your system. When you clear genetic weaknesses from your system it not only frees up your body and mind, it also clears away the weak genetic imprint for future generations in your bloodline.

Of course, in some cases the genetic imprint may be too dominant to clear in this lifetime. It could be due to your bloodline, but it also has to do with your karmic predisposition. Healing doesn't always have to mean that one is fit, healthy and full of energy. Healing also means being at peace and content with whatever challenges or joys life sends our way. Sometimes illness cannot be avoided, and in such cases the healing is in learning to be okay with the sickness. By allowing it to teach you something, you are essentially letting it help you to evolve and overcome something.

How Often to Practice?

If you are new to the technique, it is best to identify your weaker chakras as soon as you can. Once identified, it is advisable to practice the chakras balancing technique at least twice a day for two weeks to get things moving in a better direction.

It takes time for new patterns to be brought in, so it is important to keep practicing during the initial 2 – 3-week period. When there has been improvement in signs, symptoms, and general well-being, you can reduce the practice to at least once every few days. It is so simple, easy, pleasant, and completely free that it is one of those things you can do for the rest of your days to gain an energy lift, to clear your head, to relax, or just to keep everything flowing in the right direction.

Chakra Pathology

There are five states in which the function and effectiveness of the chakras can become compromised:

1. **Scrambled:** This refers to a scrambling of the electrical system of the aura through its meridians and other energy bodies. This is the most common pathology in the modern world due to excess computer usage and the consumption of sugars and stimulants.

2. **Deficient:** There is a distinct lack of energy available within the chakra for it to function properly.

3. **Excess:** There is too much energy in the chakra, and it is usually dominating, overpowering, and taxing energy from other chakras. Wherever there is an excess there must also be a deficiency in the system. The most common chakra to generate excess is the solar plexus, due to the influence of the liver and the ego.

4. **Blocked:** There is a blockage in the distribution of energy within the chakras and meridian system.

5. **Stagnant:** There is a sluggish area within the chakra system that is affecting the flow of the entire system. In this case, tonification (spinning with more circles and spinning more often) is the best remedy.

Energy in the chakra system tends to flow upwards (Kundalini). So in treatment, if you begin by treating the lower chakra first, it will then nourish and draw the energy upwards and will address and balance out the upper chakras naturally.

The Chakras

There are literally hundreds of books and resources on the internet that go into great detail and elaborate explanations of the chakras and their meanings. For this book, I am focusing more on the actual practice of chakra balancing and spinning rather than going into detailed explanations of the chakras. It is important to experience them for yourself, and not to hold too strongly onto the descriptions you find in books and other places.

Sometimes the colors may be different or the feelings may be different than what is often outlined in books. In such a case, follow your own experience and intuition first; the books just serve as a guide. But for those who are unfamiliar with the chakras, I have delved a little into each one below. Feel free to explore other books and resources on the chakras, as they all have something of value.

1st chakra / base

(pubic bone, base of torso)

This is one of the major energy stations. The 1st and 2nd chakras are the primary energy stations that feed the other chakras. Conditions like chronic fatigue and adrenal exhaustion are due to the 1st and/or 2nd chakras being deficient in energy, blocked, or totally scrambled. To be fully in the physical world and in our bodies, this chakra needs to be functioning and spinning properly. This chakra is the center of our most ancient and tribal rhythm. It is our deepest connection to mother earth. It is our earthing rod, essentially, that grounds out any excess electro activity that we may have picked up throughout the day. It helps us to ground, stabilize and unscramble. It calms the mind and provides us with a deep sense of inner strength and confidence. This is the chakra of drumming, of music, of dance, of primary urges — to run, jump, dance, sing and mate.

2nd chakra / womb / dan tien

(About one inch below the navel)

This is the chakra of our truest potential — a womb-like center that carries our gifts and our wisdom through various lifetimes. When we are walking our soul's true path this chakra is alive, strong and powerful. It feeds us with great confidence and courage. It is strongly connected to our primal fire — our fire for life, to experience life, to share life, to create life, to support life; hence its connection to the mother/baby energy of nourishment and support. This chakra centre is also our powerhouse. If this area is functioning well, our overall energy field, our state of mind, and the health of our entire system will be strong and positively influential. It is also where our internal energies are stored for later life.

3rd chakra / solar plexus

(About one inch below the bottom of the sternum in the fleshy area of the upper belly)

This is a very active and often volatile energy center. It is the chakra that expresses the ego, or in other words, the identification of oneself and one's individuality. It is a powerful center that extends itself easily out into the world. It likes to express itself through movement, through intelligence and through social connections. If this chakra is dysfunctional or unbalanced it often leads to egocentric behavior, anger, rage, frustration, nausea, digestive problems and toxic overload in the liver. In the local area of the solar plexus reside many organs, and this chakra helps to regulate these organs, namely the liver, gallbladder, stomach and spleen.

4th chakra / heart

(In the center of the chest and sternum)

The heart chakra is the chakra of love, compassion, and being able to feel and sense the nature of others. When it is balanced you feel open to life, open to new people, and accepting of the world as it is. When the heart chakra is functioning well, you tend to feel your way through life rather than overthinking, over-planning, or trying to intellectualize everything. When the heart chakra is out of balance, there is a real difficulty in relating to others, in accepting others, and in feeling forgiveness or compassion. In some cases there is a real "hate" that exists, and this is harmful, mostly to the actual person who is doing the "hating". If something annoys you or frustrates you, the best thing you can do is open your heart and just let it in – then it won't bother you anymore. Try it.

5*th chakra / throat*

(At the base of the neck, sitting in the grove of the upper sternum) — thyroid gland

The throat chakra is the center of communication and it has a lot to do with speaking our truth. The throat chakra is almost always deficient or blocked in most people. I think this is largely due to the western, mainly English-style culture of choosing politeness and avoidance of awkward situations rather than speaking up or confronting someone. When this chakra is under stress the tone of the voice can be weak, excessively loud, wavering, or simply harsh to the ear. When this chakra is balanced and working well, the tone of the voice is soothing and comforting and has a healthy and balancing effect on all those who hear it. It is especially important for this area to be balanced if you use your voice for your work life, e.g. if you are a teacher, phone consultant, presenter, singer, etc.

6*th chakra / third eye*

(Between the eyebrows)

This is the center of the intellect and of intuition. When this chakra is balanced, great ideas, inventions, and intuitions can easily be received. It is like an opening for great insight and inspiration that allows for rapid personal and spiritual evolution. When this area is out of balance it often leads to regular headaches, foggy head, eye problems, sinus problems and a real lack of intuition and inspiration. It can be put out of balance through excessive thinking which affects the whole system, or, on the other end of the spectrum, under-thinking, most commonly due to dulling the mind with intoxicants and sedative drugs. This tends to lead to a real lack of inspiration in the person, and often leads to one feeling increasingly lost and depressed, as their ability to tap into their intuition has been compromised.

7th chakra / top of head

(Top of the head)

This is the chakra of highest spiritual truth. This centre essentially connects us with all that is — with the universe and each other. It provides us also with great insight and intuition. When balanced it also brings us a heightened state of energy and a feeling of being protected by the universe; a sense of faith becomes increasingly present. When this chakra is blocked or unbalanced there is an increased feeling of being alone in the world. The mind can easily become dull or overcritical and judgmental of the world because it has come to shut itself off from its higher knowledge.

The Most Common Problem Activities in Our Modern World

1. Too much time sitting with poor posture in badly designed furniture (the knees need to be positioned slightly lower than the hips when seated, as this supports the correct tilt of the pelvis and hips).

2. Overstimulation of mind and eyes through computer work, computer games, mobile computer devices, movies and digital entertainment. Ideally, no more than four hours a day of computer-based work.

3. Overuse and reliance on stimulant drinks, caffeine, drugs (including pharmaceuticals) and alcohol.

4. Too much sugar, white bread, dairy, and processed fatty foods. Yes, we all know it...

5. Not enough movement of the body in general. Lack of exercise (The body is designed to move). Walking can be enough!

6. Overthinking; excess worry. Please, don't take your thoughts too seriously; there is much more to you than just your thinking mind. There is a time to think and there is a time to just be. The mind will always churn out thoughts and images, but you don't have to give it your attention. Find the balance between listening to the mind when you need it and "turning it down" by placing your attention somewhere else when you don't

want or need to think. (For more information on meditation, check out my other book "Mediation Made Simple".)

7. Putting too much pressure and expectation on yourself and others. This will eventually lead to other stresses and drain all your energy systems. If you push too hard, it is likely that you will eventually slingshot yourself to the other spectrum and become adrenally fatigued. This can lead to chronic fatigue syndrome, depression, etc. Nature moves slowly and patiently, and rests often.

8. Unsupportive and abusive relationships.

More Advanced Techniques

The following are techniques for those interested in utilizing applied kinesiology. If you find the following too difficult or confusing then don't worry about it, and just stick to what we have already covered. What we have already covered is just as effective and powerful as these other techniques I will be discussing.

Applied kinesiology consists of "muscle testing", and was first discovered and developed in the 1970s. When we muscle test, we are receiving direct feedback from the body itself and bypassing the conscious mind. It takes time and practice to develop the sensitivity to it, but once you have got it worked out it is an invaluable tool. Modern science tends to ridicule the muscle testing procedure but this is simply because it is not fully understood. Muscle testing is not just testing body function; it is also moving into the world of subtle energetics. The energetic realm is not fully understood by science yet, so until it is, it will continue to be ridiculed in most medicine circles. All great discoveries tend to take at least 30 – 50 years before they get accepted as common practice and common knowledge.

I will provide a basic overview of the procedure here, but if you want more information and more experience with muscle testing then it is best to receive more formal education. The system of "Touch for Health" (Google it) is a good place to start, and they offer the training all over the world.

Okay, so this is how you do it:

1. Bring the extended arm of the patient to the side of their body, with their palm facing outwards.

2. Start from the base chakra and tap the chakra area with a little tap to indicate to the body that this is what we want to test. Straight after tapping, place your fingers gently above their wrist and try to draw the patient's arm away and out to the side while the patient gently resists. About two pounds of pressure is enough.

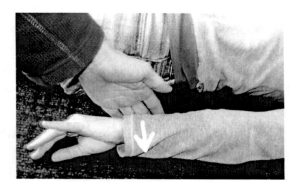

3. If the arm is strong and it is difficult to move then this indicates that the chakra is strong, "switched on", and functioning well. Move on to the next chakra and test using step 2.

4. When the arm tests as weak, meaning that it is easy to draw the arm away from the body, then this indicates the chakra is not functioning well and is "switched

off". When this is the case, begin to spin the chakra in question. Simply bring your palm above the chakra in the area of focus and begin circling your hand and arm in a counterclockwise direction, like spinning a vinyl record on a record player. You can circle your hand close to the body to begin with; there is no need to touch the body with this technique. You can then draw the palm away from the body while continuing to circle it. You can vary the distance from the body as much as you like or feel is appropriate. Most people feel warmth, or something like a dense, misty air with their palms while spinning. Spin for 1 – 5 minutes.

5. Next, shake your hands off, rub the hands together to neutralize any electrical charge, and begin spinning in the same area, this time in a clockwise direction. Again, you can vary the distance from the body as you much as you like and feel is appropriate. Spin for 1 – 3 minutes (usually a little less then counterclockwise).

6. Now you can focus on the next chakra that has come to your attention with muscle testing. When you find a weak chakra, repeat 4 – 5.

7. Continue until all seven chakras are functioning well. There will likely be a noticeable difference in the patient's state, e.g. clearer eyes, being more relaxed, less pain, etc. Finish with a sip of water and a deep breath for both patient and practitioner.

Working on Particular Issues or Stresses

This practice involves more applied kinesiology techniques.

1. Ask the patient to bring a particular issue of stress to the mind. Saying it out loud is recommended as it makes it more present and clear in the mind, e.g. "I feel stressed out by my boss at work", "I'm confused about my life", "Every time I think about . . . I feel anxious".

2. Soon after stating the issue, get the patient to bring their legs together and then bring them comfortably apart, so the feet are roughly 20 – 30 centimeters away from each other. Once they have moved in this way it's important that they don't move their legs again until the chakra balancing is complete. Instruct them not to move their legs until the chakra spinning is over. This movement holds the energy of the issue "in circuit" within the hips and legs so that it can be worked on. If they are to move the legs, the energy containing the issue at hand will disperse and be released.

3. Either begin muscle testing to locate the malfunctioning chakras, or just go through all of them step by step beginning at the base chakra and moving upwards. Questioning can also help to identify weak parts of the body as discussed earlier.

4. Every time a malfunctioning chakra is located, simply bring your palm above the chakra in the area of focus

and begin circling your hand and arm in a counterclockwise direction, like spinning a vinyl record on a record player. You can circle your hand close to the body to begin with; there is no need to touch the body with this technique. You can then draw the palm away from the body while continuing to circle it. You can vary the distance from the body as much as you like or feel is appropriate. Most people feel warmth, or something like a dense, misty air with their palms while spinning. Spin for 1 – 5 minutes.

5. Next, shake your hands off, rub the hands together to neutralize any electrical charge, and begin spinning in the same area, this time in a clockwise direction. Again, you can vary the distance from the body as you much as you like and feel is appropriate. Spin for 1 – 3 minutes (usually a little less then counterclockwise).

6. Now you can focus on the next chakra that has come to your attention with muscle testing. When you find a weak chakra, repeat steps 4 – 5.

7. Continue until all seven chakras are functioning well. There will likely be a noticeable difference in the patient's state, e.g. clearer eyes, being more relaxed, less pain, etc. Finish with a sip of water and a deep breath for both patient and practitioner.

Other Effective Ways to Balance the Chakras

Chakra spinning is not the only way to get the chakras to function optimally. A variety of practices like yoga asana, some exercises, breathing regulation, meditation, acupuncture, herbal medicine, energy medicine and a supportive diet can assist in the overall function of the body and chakra system. Take time to relax and centre yourself throughout the day. Here are some simple ideas:

- Go for a gentle walk. Don't add more stress to your body by carrying mobile computer devices and jamming ear buds into your ears and listening to loud music. Reduce the input! Just walk, be present, feel your feet, smell the air, listen to the birds. There is plenty going on already, do you really need to add more "noise" to your system?

- Lie down for fifteen minutes. Close your eyes and rest. Let thoughts pass through you; don't place any importance on them for this fifteen minutes. Give yourself permission to let them go. You can always deal with those thoughts later if they are so important. Don't take your thoughts too seriously.

- Cross your legs, interlace your fingers, close your eyes and relax for 10 – 15 minutes. Interlacing our limbs by crossing the left and right sides of our bodies allows our energetics to restore and rebalance themselves.

Sitting cross-legged on the floor for a few minutes can really change the way you feel.

- Chakra meditation. You can balance the chakras through the mind using a mantra. This is a technique that deserves more time and explanation. Therefore, I will write about this in more detail in another book to come out soon.

Final Words

Hopefully by now you have come to see that chakra balancing is a very simple, easy and effective technique that anyone can practice. It is not meant to be complicated, and it does not require any special knowledge, skills or materials to be able to practice it— just intention and a willingness to participate. We can all do it. We all have the capacity to balance the chakras.

This technique can help to lessen the gap of feeling powerless when our loved ones and friends become ill. We can use this technique to become more helpful and make a difference to those who are sick or just need a little boost throughout their day. Simple things like chakra balancing can make a big difference to the well-being of ourselves and of others.

~ May All Beings Be Happy ~

Other Titles by Michael Hetherington

How to Do Restorative Yoga

The Little Book of Yin

How to Learn Acupuncture

Moving From Our Head to Our Heart

The Art of Muscle Testing

CPSIA information can be obtained
at www.ICGtesting.com
Printed in the USA
LVOW08s0956011116
511034LV00047B/1373/P